3D Printing of Medical Models from CT-MRI Images

A Practical step-by-step guide

3D Printing of Medical Models from CT-MRI Images
A Practical step-by-step guide

Li Yihua, Eric Luis

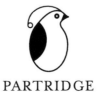

PARTRIDGE

ISBN: Hardcover   978-1-4828-7941-4
             Softcover   978-1-4828-7940-7
             eBook   978-1-4828-7942-1

To order additional copies of this book, contact
Toll Free 800 101 2657 (Singapore)
Toll Free 1 800 81 7340 (Malaysia)
orders.singapore@partridgepublishing.com

www.partridgepublishing.com/singapore

Foreword

3D Printing is leading the next industrial revolution. President Obama has called 3D Printing: "the potential to revolutionize" in his State of the Union Address in February, 2013. Following that, healthcare providers, medical device makers, biopharmaceuticals, third-party payers, educational institutions are all jumping onto the 3D printing wagon.

The Brigham and Women's Hospital in Boston has used 3D printers to assist with face transplants and the Shriners Hospital for Children in Houston, Texas, has used 3D printing to create prosthetic hands for kids. The 3D printed head and hand models allow doctors to explain to patients more clearly, perform pre-operative planning and practise on models prior to the actual surgeries to achieve greater accuracy.

Medical Schools and teaching institutions have also found 3D printed anatomical models to be extremely useful for anatomy dissection, pathology, surgery and other clinical subspecialties.

It will be ideal, therefore, for all medical students, clinical specialists and all related personnel in the healthcare industry to be introduced and equipped with the various skills and resources in 3D Printing available to them.

This first instructional manual "3D-Printing of Medical Models from CT-MRI" images has been very nicely written to bridge the gap from CT-MRI films to the 3D Printers. The practical step-by-step approach will help readers quickly grasp the essence of converting CT-MRI DICOM images to STL (stereolithograhic) files, which are ready for 3D printing.

I hope all our readers will benefit from this book and continue to explore your 3D printing adventures.

Professor Chee Kai CHUA

Executive Director, Singapore Center for 3D Printing
Professor, School of Mechanical and Aerospace Engineering, Nanyang Technological University

Contents

Chapter 1 Introduction..1

    1.1 Why print 3D models from CT or MRI scans? 3

    1.2 General concept 4

Chapter 2 Preparing the DICOM dataset 7

    2.1 Introduction to 3D slicer 9

    2.2 User interface..9

    2.3 Importing your dataset.....................................12

    2.4 Generating the 3D visualization........................15

    2.5 Analyzing the dataset......................................18

    2.6 Isolating the region of interest (ROI).................21

    2.7 Cropping the ROI...23

Chapter 3 Creating the 3D volume (Segmentation) 25

    3.1 Editor module...27

    3.2 Managing Label maps 28

    3.3 Editing Selected Label Map 29

    3.4 Creating the 3D model 34

    3.5 Scene management...35

    3.6 Comparing the result..37

    3.7 Analyzing the problem 38

3.8 Patching the label map (Wand Effect) 40

3.9 Patching the label map (Manual painting).............................. 43

3.10 Saving and loading your progress 45

3.11 Exporting the model... 50

Chapter 4 Other Tools 55

Exploring other tools.. 57

4.1 Identify Island Effect: 58

4.2 Change Island Effect: 60

4.3 Remove Islands Effect: 61

4.4 Save Island Effect:... 63

4.5 Erode and Dilate Effect 64

4.6 Grow Cut and Watershed from Markers Effect 64

4.7 Change Label Effect 65

4.8 Fast Marching Effect 67

Moving on.. 69

Chapter 5 Preparing for printing 71

5.1 Introduction to Autodesk Meshmixer 73

5.2 User interface.. 73

5.3 Reducing the triangle count.. 75

5.4 Plane cut 78

5.5 Further cleaning 80

5.6 Fixing flaws from the segmentation 82

5.7 Bridging gaps 84

4.8 Preparing for print 86

Chapter 6 Conclusion 91

6.1 Acknowledgements 93

CHAPTER 1

Introduction

This instructional book is written for beginners to help bridge the gap between CT/MRI radiological images and 3D printing of medical models. The programs we utilize in this book are available for free, and suitable for beginners.

We have incorporated only the basic segmentation techniques to help you get started. Our aim is to introduce to you the concept of 3D segmentation, and how that translates into a 3-dimensional model that can be 3D-printed.

With this foundation, we hope you will embark on the adventurous journey of 3D printing and discover new arenas.

Yihua Li, Eric Luis.

1.1 Why print 3D models from CT or MRI scans?

In operative surgeries, 3d printed models are used for pre-operative planning, pre-operative surgical skills training for surgeons and surgical residents, thus improving surgical outcomes.

In clinical practices, conferences and seminars, presenters can put across ideas in a much clearer fashion, improving the interaction and understanding of difficult concepts and topics.

In anatomy or pathology labs, 3D printed models can substitute for real models, owing to paucity of the real specimens. Repeated dissection of the same anatomical regions can be performed.

In medical schools or art institutions, 3D printed models are used for teaching and designing purposes.

3D printed models can assist patients and caregivers with decision-making and giving informed consent and improving patient satisfaction.

1.2 General concept

Before we begin, I would like to bring you through the workflow, and get a rough idea of the general concept. For the total beginner, you might not get the full grasp on the first read of the work flow. But you will get a better grip of the concept as you work through the rest of the book, armed with this general knowledge.

1- What is in a dataset?

A dataset is a collection of images. They usually come in, but is not limited to, DICOM format. In our case, the images are slices from a CT/MRI scan, usually in axial plane.

2- Data analysis with Volume Rendering

When we import the dataset, the program reads the images, and generates the sagittal and coronal views. Giving us a total of 3 anatomical views.

Before we can generate the 3D model for 3D printing, I recommend doing a quick render with Volume Rendering. This will allow us to better plan our steps ahead.

Volume Rendering stacks the dataset, applies color and opacity over it to generate a **'pseudo-3D' image**. This image gives us a very good preview of what the actual 3D image will look like and helps us identify potential problems we might encounter later.

3- Create Label Map

A **Label Map** is the building block for our 3D model. Like how a 2D image is built from pixels (left), a Label Map is a 3D volume built from voxels (Right). This is then used to generate the tangible 3D volume we can print.

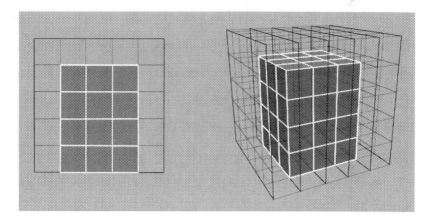

4- Make Model

Once we have clean **Label Maps**, we can generate good 3D models from them.

5- Clean up

Make Model is a very basic tool to create the 3D model, but the advantage of it is that it does not leave out any details. However it also includes all the noise. We will go through various techniques to clean up the model.

CHAPTER 2

Preparing the DICOM dataset

2.1 Introduction to 3D slicer

3D Slicer is an open source software available on multiple operating systems. It allows for the analysis and visualization of medical images; and most importantly, for the interest of this book, generate 3D volumes that can be used for 3D printing.

2.2 User interface

For the purpose of this tutorial, we will only touch on some of the basic tools. Detailed documentation of its tools and plug-ins are available on its official website.

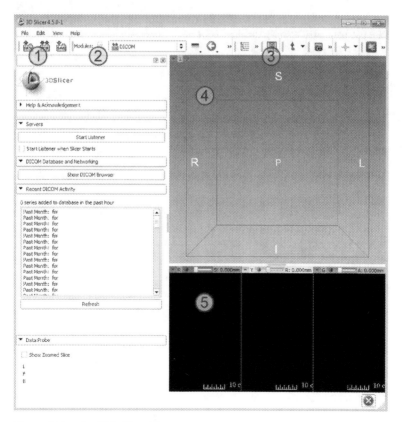

Figure 1 Standard 3D Slicer UI

1: Add data allows you to add individual DICOM sequences to the existing scene.

DICOM browser calls up the DICOM browser window that allows you to load you dataset of interest into the scene.

Save the scene and/or export your segmentation.

2: **Module Panel** allows you to search for modules to perform different operations on the dataset.

3: Choose from a list of default **Layout** settings

4: Your 3D renders appears in this **3D viewport**.

Left mouse click + drag: Rotates camera.

Ctrl + Left mouse click + drag: Rotates camera on one axis.

Shift + Left mouse click +drag /Middle mouse click + drag: Camera pan.

Middle mouse roller/ Right mouse click + drag: Camera zoom.

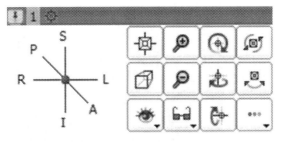

Figure 2 Extra display options for the 3D work space

Mouse-over the pin to show extra display option for the viewport. Click to pin the viewport. You can mouse-over the extra icons to display their functions.

1 :Displays the name of the viewport. (First 3D view.)

:Centers the 3D model on the viewport.

5:

Slice Viewer displays the slices of your dataset in **Axial, Sagittal** and **Coronal** planes.

Left mouse click + Drag: Changes the value contrast of your slides.

Middle mouse roller: Allows you to move through the slices.

Middle mouse click + drag: Camera pan.

Right mouse click + drag: Camera zoom.

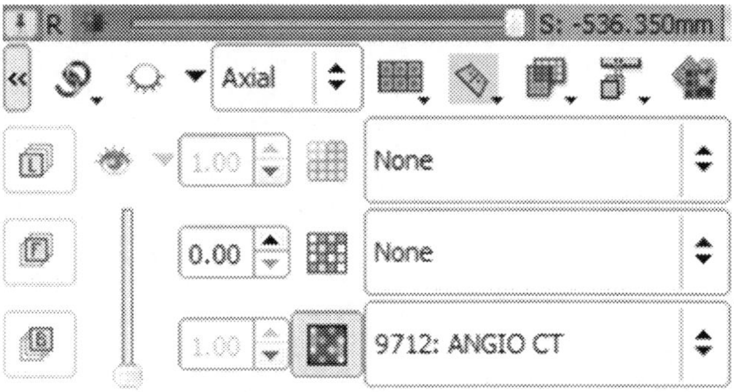

Figure 3 Extra display options for the Slice viewer

Mouse-over the pin to show extra option for the viewport. Click on it to pin the viewport. You can mouse-over the extra icons to display their functions.

R :Name of the viewport. (R= Red, Y= Yellow, G= Green)

■ :Centers the slice in the viewport.

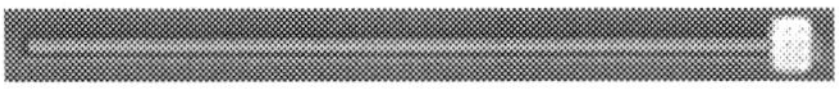

▬▬▬▬▬▬▬ :Slide to move through the slices.

2.3 Importing your dataset

For the first example, we will be using ANGIO CT for MANIX. You can download the dataset from http://www.osirix-viewer.com/datasets/

Once you run **3DSlicer**, a default window like that of *Figure 1* should appear. Click on 🗠 (DICOM browser) to bring up the browser window.

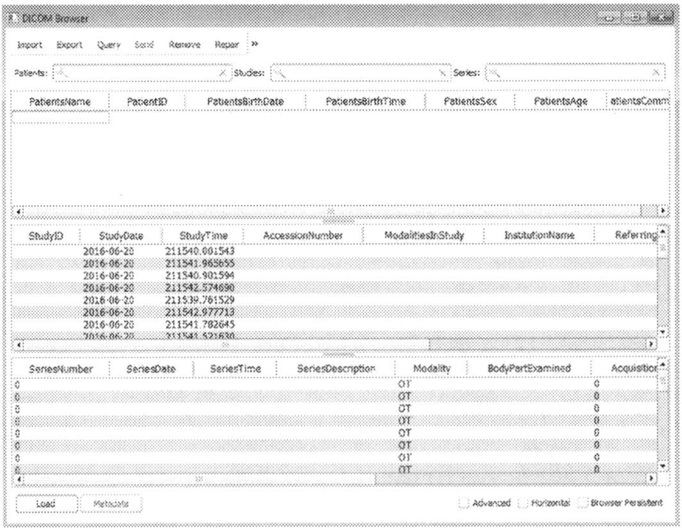

Figure 4 DICOM browser window

Click on the **Import** button, locate the folder where your DICOM sequence is stored in, select the folder, and click **Import** *on the new window.*

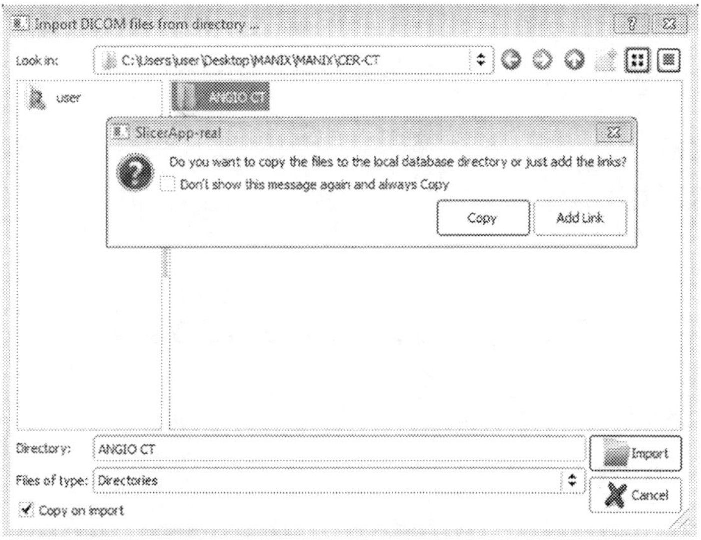

Figure 5 Copying dataset onto local database

After which, a window will pop up, asking if you would like to copy your dataset to the local database. Click copy.

You should see the following window when the import is successful. Click **OK** to proceed.

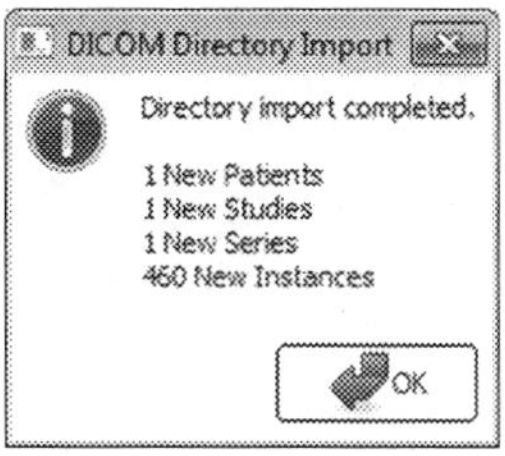

Figure 6 Import successful!

In your DICOM browser window, a new line of text should appear in each sub-window, showing details of the case study.

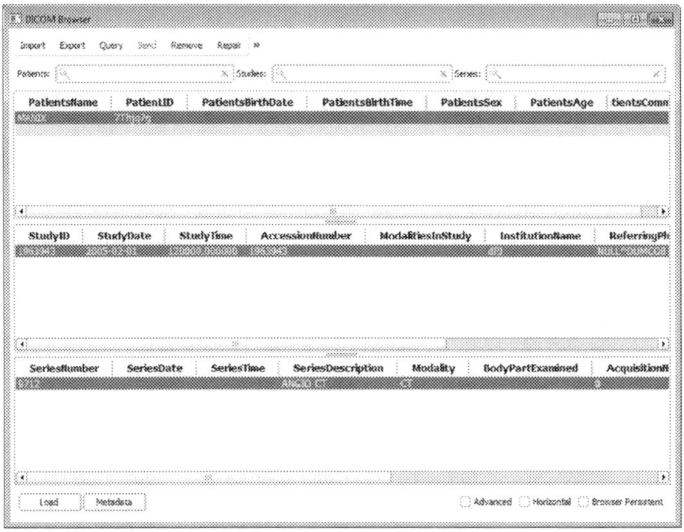

Figure 7 Imported dataset appears on the browser

Select the dataset of interest, and click Load. This process can take some time, depending on the size of your dataset.

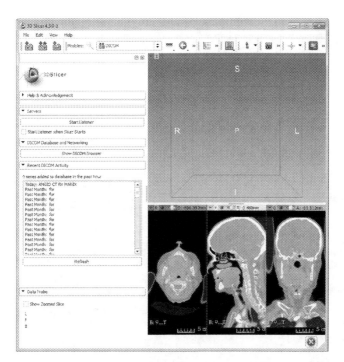

Figure 8 Dataset loaded will appear in the Slice Viewer windows

Now that the dataset is loaded into 3D slicer, we are ready to analyze the images.

2.4 Generating the 3D visualization

Click on the ![Modules: DICOM] (Module Panel) to drop down the list of modules and look for the Volume Rendering module (*Figure 10*).

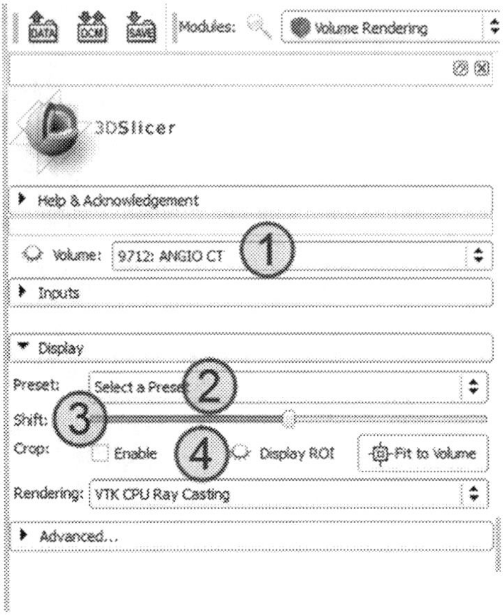

Figure 9 Volume Rendering module properties

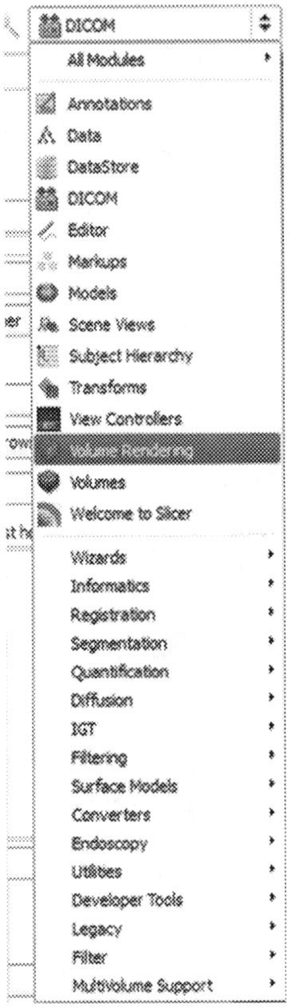

Figure 10 Volume rendering module

1- **Volume**: Select a volume from the drop-down menu to render. Click on the eye logo on the left to toggle visibility.

2- **Preset**: Choose from a set of pre-defined functions for the opacity, color and gradient transfer. You might have to tune it manually to fit your data.

3- **Shift**: This shifts the transfer data of your current preset. *(This will be explained in detail later.)*

4- **ROI**: This allow you to isolate the region of interest. Click on the eye logo on the left to toggle visibility. *(This will be explained in further detail later.)*

After you load the Volume Rendering module, its parameters will appear in the left panel *(Figure 9).*

The Volume Rendering module is a built-in module that generates an interactive 3D visualization from the dataset. By analyzing the 3D volume, we are able to access the quality of the dataset.

Turn on the visibility of the **Volume** parameter and choose the dataset of interest.

Under the **Preset** parameter, choose a preset that matches your dataset. In this case, the **CT-Bones** preset is close enough; since we are interested in segmenting the skull.

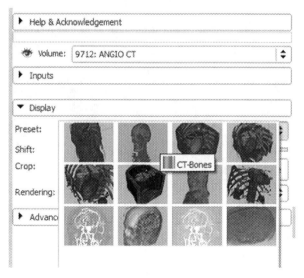

Figure 11 Choosing a render preset

Once you chose a preset *(and if the volume visibility is turned on)*, the computer will generate the 3D visualization in the background. Wait patiently, as this process can take up to a few minutes, depending on the scale of the dataset.

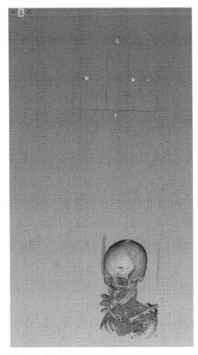

Figure 12

While the 3D image is being generated, you can still adjust the 3D viewport. Mouse over the 3D viewport and roll the middle mouse button to zoom out. Chances are, the generated 3D image is far off-center, as shown in *(Figure12)*.

Click on the Center 3D view button to snap the volume to the center of the 3D space. *(Figure 13)*.

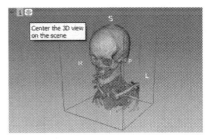

Figure 13

2.5 Analyzing the dataset

By manipulating the range slider under the **Shift** parameter, we are able to influence the transfer function. This changes the amount of details that will be rendered.

Under the **Advanced...** tab, you can have additional control over the threshold of the transfer function by manipulating the control points on the ramp under **Scalar Opacity Mapping**.

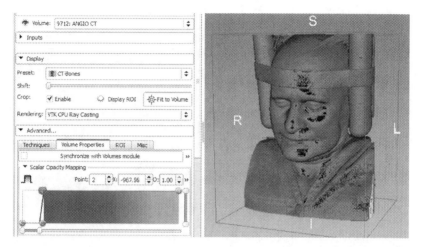

Figure 14 Shift on low

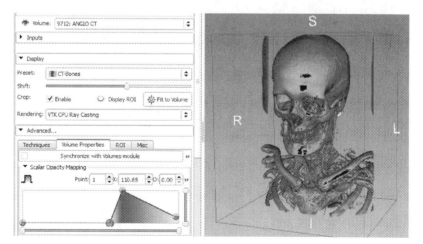

Figure 15 Shift on high

Different settings will yield vastly different results, *Figure 14* and *Figure 15* are more extreme example of such. By scrubbing through the Shift parameter quickly, we can get a good gauge of the quality of the dataset we are working with.

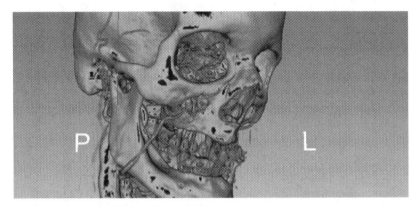

Figure 16 A closer look at the volume render

By analyzing the 3D render, we can more or less anticipate potential problems with the volume that we will generate later for 3D printing.

We can see that the alveolar processes, infra-orbital foramen, nasal cavity and interior of the eye socket are either noisy or missing. This is largely because the dataset is originally a CT angiogram, so the blood vessels tend to get in the way. However, we will look at how we can try to rectify these problems later on.

2.6 Isolating the region of interest (ROI)

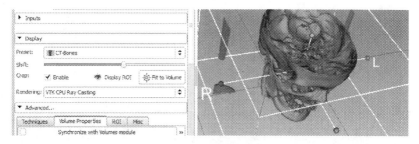

Figure 17 Using the ROI function to see the interior of the skull

Toggle on the **Display ROI** parameter by clicking on the eye.

A cube will appear around the 3D volume. On each plane of the cube is a ball-shaped handle that you can click and drag to cut out the unwanted regions.

Having the planes cut into the volume will allow you to see cross sections of the model.

At this point, you are still able to go back and adjust the **Shift** and **Scalar Opacity Mapping** parameters to analyze the interior surfaces.

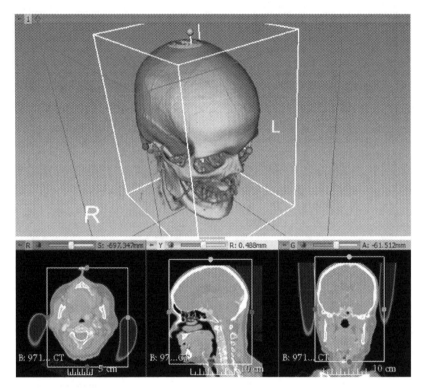

Figure 18 Define the ROI to crop

You may also use the handles in the Slice Viewer to crop the 3D volume.

Now that we have decided on the region we want to use, we can crop out the other regions. This is helpful if your ROI is only a small part of the scan. A heavy volume takes up unnecessary computing power and slows down your work.

2.7 Cropping the ROI

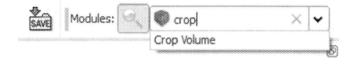

Figure 19 Searching for the **Crop Volume** module

Search for the **Crop Volume** module from the module list. It should load up the Crop Volume parameters on the module panel.

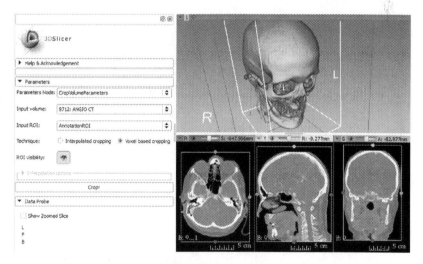

Figure 20 Crop Volume module properties

Check the **Voxel based cropping** option and click **Crop!**

In the Slice Viewer window, you should see that the DICOM slices are cropped according to your defined ROI.

Before moving on, I recommend turning off the visibility of the volume render. This might get in the way in later steps.

Conclusion

The Volume Rendering module generates a 3D visualization from the DICOM sequence. This 3D volume, however, cannot be used for printing. The visualization is only a gauge for us to anticipate any problems we might face with the actual 3D volume that we will generate, and determine the quality of the dataset.

After the analysis, we are ready to move on to create the actual 3D volume that can be used for printing.

CHAPTER 3

Creating the 3D volume (Segmentation)

3.1 Editor module

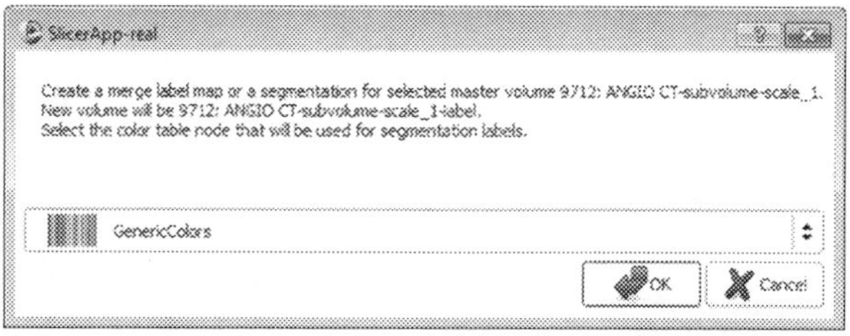

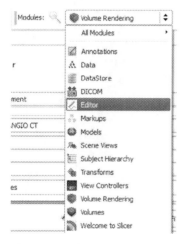

Figure 21 Selecting a colour table for your label map

Figure 22 Editor module

The **Editor** module allows you to create and edit label maps, which the 3D volume will be based off.

Once you select the Editor module from the module list, a pop-up window appears, prompting you to choose a color table node to be used for the segmentation. (*Figure 21*)

The color table is merely a color code for your label map, you may choose any set from the list. For this tutorial, we will use **Generic Colors**.

Click **OK** and proceed.

3.2 Managing Label maps

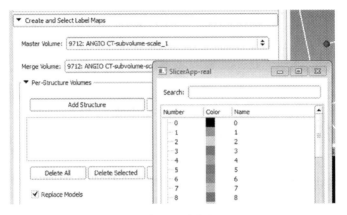

Figure 23 Choosing a colour for your label map

Under **Per-Structure Volumes** tab, click **Add Structure**. A window appears, prompting you to choose a color code for your label map. Choose a color that will stand out against the black background of the Slice Viewer and white areas of the dataset.

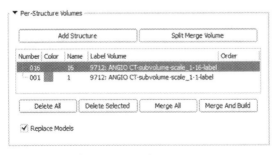

Figure 24 Label maps created

Once the label map is created, it will be listed under **Per-Structure Volumes**. You can have as many labels as you like, each one segmenting different regions, then either merge them into one singe volume, or create individual models from each label map.

3.3 Editing Selected Label Map

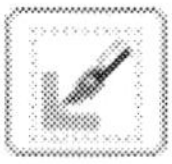

Paint effect:

Click and drag to paint your label map on the Slice Viewer.

-**Threshold paint**: Applies threshold on your strokes. Use the slider to adjust threshold value.

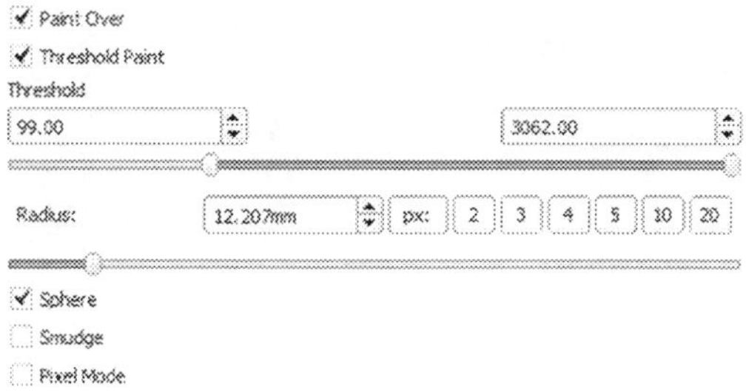

Figure 25 Paint Effect properties

-**Radius**:   Enter values, pick from default sizes or use the slider to adjust brush radius.

-**Sphere**: Makes the brush a sphere, your strokes will affect multiple layers.

-**Smudge**: Alters the boundaries of your label map.

-Pixel Mode: Paints exactly one pixel where you click.

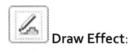 **Draw Effect**:

Click to create straight lines between points. Use the 'x' key to delete the last point added. Click and drag to draw curves.

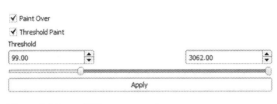

Figure 26 Draw Effect properties

Draw the outline of the region you want to add to your label map. Right click or use 'a' key to apply.

-**Threshold Paint**: Applies threshold on your region. Use the slider to adjust threshold value.

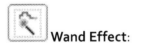 **Wand Effect**:

Fills connected regions with similar intensities. Clicking multiple time will grow the region.

Figure 27 Wand Effect properties

-**Tolerance**: Controls the sensitivity of the fill at picking out similar pixels.

-**Max Pixels per click**: Controls the area covered with each click.

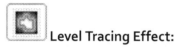

Figure 28 Adjusting the range for the **Threshold**

-**Fill Volume**: When checked, the fill grows in 3D, across layers.

-**Threshold Paint**: Similar to the Tolerance attribute. Adjust sensitivity through the range slider.

Level Tracing Effect:

Selects an entire connected region of similar value. Region gets highlighted when mouse pointer hovers over the region. Left click to apply region.

-**Threshold Paint**: Controls the sensitivity of the region select when picking similar pixels.

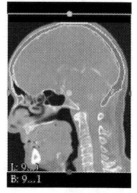

Figure 29 Region selected with **Level Tracing Effect**

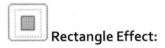 **Rectangle Effect:**

Left click and drag to draw rectangle. Release to apply selected region.

-**Threshold paint**: applied threshold effect within the drawn region.

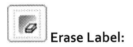 **Erase Label:**

Erase label can be activated on top of the above mentioned tools. When toggled on, the previous tool works in reverse; erases rather than add to the label map.

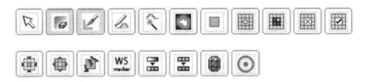

Figure 30 Using **Erase Label** over the **Paint Effect**

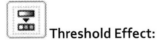 **Threshold Effect:**

This selects similar pixels across the entire dataset.

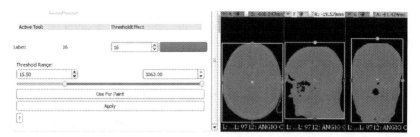

Figure 31 Default setting for **Threshold Effect**

Once you activate **Threshold Effect** tool, the regions of similar value on the dataset will be highlighted in the color label. The region should now be flashing; indicating that you have not applied the effect.

-**Threshold Range**: Use the range sliders to define the range of values that you want to be highlighted. Different values can give vastly different results. Compare *Figure 31* and *Figure 32*. Play around with the range to achieve a best fit result. If a scan is high quality and sharp. The label map generated should be relatively clean too.

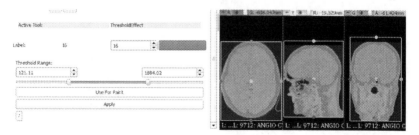

Figure 32 Refined **Threshold Range**

-**Use For Paint**: Transfer the current threshold setting to be used for other labeling operations such as Paint or Draw.

Scrub through the layers on the **Slice Viewer** to check the generated label map. While scrubbing through, you are still able to adjust your Threshold Range.

Once you are happy with the result. Click **Apply**. The flashing in the **Slice Viewer** should stop; indicating that the label map has been created.

3.4 Creating the 3D model

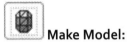 **Make Model:**

Make Model generates a 3D object form the selected label map. This 3D object can then be exported into printable formats.

Active Tool:		MakeModelEffect	
Label:	1	1	

Go To Model Maker

✔ Smooth Model

Model Name: 1

Apply

Figure 33 Make Model properties

-**Model Name**: Name the model that will be generated. This is recommended if you are doing multiple segmentations within the same scene, for ease of management.

-**Apply**: The model-building runs in the background. It might take some time, depending on the scale and complexity of the segmentation. Once done, the model will appear in the 3D viewport.

-Smooth Model: Having this option on will apply a smooth on the generated model. The result looks better, but will be heavier on the computer, hence, takes longer. Below is a comparison of a smoothed and unsmoothed model.

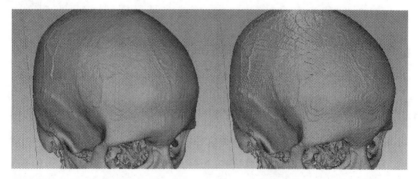

Figure 34 Left: Smoothed model. Right: Unsmoothed model

3.5 Scene management

At this stage, the generated model might not be of the best quality. Unfortunately, unlike **Volume Rendering**, the model will not update live automatically as we adjust the **Threshold Range** on the label map. We can delete this model and start over from creating a new label map, until you obtain a satisfactory result.

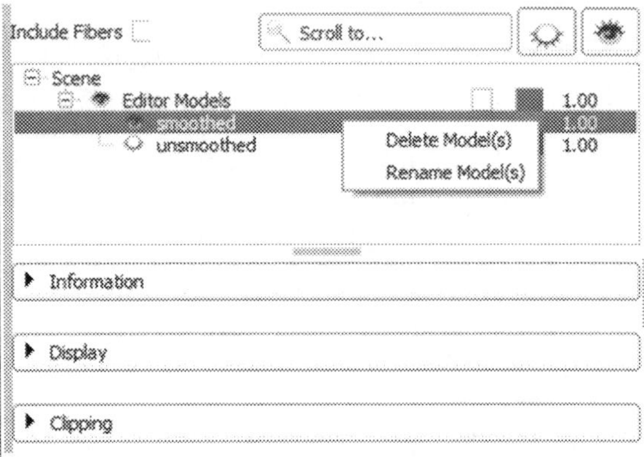

Figure 35 Delete/ Rename option

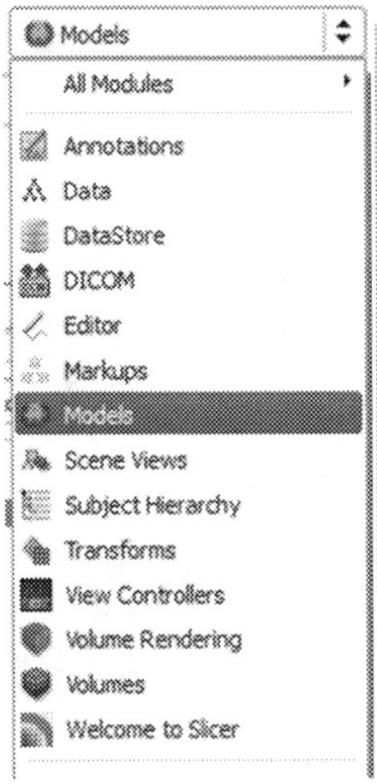

Figure 36 Models module

Using the **Models** module, we can effectively manage our scene, as we experiment with the label map to achieve a good model.

In the **Scroll to...** box, you can key in the name of the model to search for it. This is helpful when you have many models in a single scene.

-Scene: All the models we have created are listed under Editor Models. Clicking on the eye icon toggles its visibility. Right clicking on the model will open up options to delete or rename the model.

The swatch on the right indicates the color of the model. Double click on it to bring up the Select Color window. You may select from the table of default colors or define you own from the color chart. This change will not be reflected on the label map.

The number on the far right is the value for its opacity. Double click on it to open up the range slider.

-Information: This tab contains properties about the selected model, such as surface area and volume.

-Display: The various sub-tabs allows you to control how the selected model is displayed within the scene.

-Clipping: Controls the clipping properties for this model.

3.6 Comparing the result

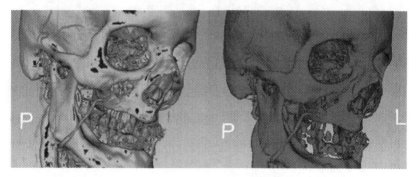

Figure 37 Left: Volume render. Right: Model generated from Model maker

Comparing the results, we can see that the visualization turned out to be quite accurate. The problems with the alveolar processes, infra-orbital foramen, nasal cavity and interior of the eye socket that we predicted using **Volume Rendering** showed up in the model generated by **Model Maker**.

3.7 Analyzing the problem

There are multiple ways to go about patching the label map. You can use the tools (Draw, Paint, Wand, Rectangle, etc.) in any combination to suit your needs. This tutorial will direct you the fastest way to patch up the label map.

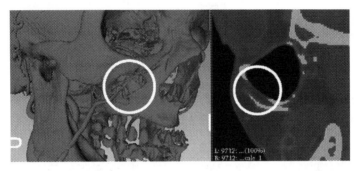

Figure 38 Identifying the hole on the model from the **Slice Viewer**

Taking a closer look at the infra-orbital foramen area of the dataset, we can roughly see where the problem lies. Due to the thinness of that particular area of the maxillary bone, it appears to have lower intensity compared to other regions. Hence, it was difficult for the Model Maker to pick out the region without also selecting other unwanted regions of similar low intensity.

In *Figure 38*, the gap in the label map (right) corresponds to the hole on the maxillary area (left).

We will attempt to fill the gap and remove the blood vessel by editing the label map, and rebuilding the model from it.

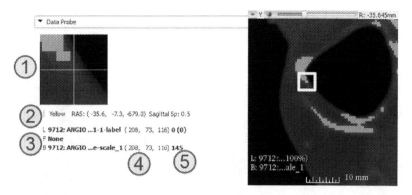

Figure 39 Data Probe

Data Probe: This tab appears at the bottom of the module panel in every module. It displays the properties of the point your mouse is on when it is within the Slice Viewer.

1- **Show Zoomed Slice**: When you turn this on, a small window pops up under the Data Probe tab whenever your mouse pointer is within the Slice Viewer. The window displays a magnified view of the point your point rests on. In this case it corresponds to the region in the white box on the **Slice Viewer**.

2- This line indicates the Slicer Viewer you are in. The color corresponds to the color of the window on the Slice Viewer. (Yellow in this case.)

Co-ordinates in the bracket reflect to the position of the pointer in the 3D viewport.

Sagittal: Refers to the orientation of the slice your pointer is on.

Sp: 0.5 refers to the spacing between each slice.

3- **L**, **F** and **B** refers to the layers in the slice viewer. They are **L**abel, **F**oreground and **B**ackground respectively. Refer to *Figure 3*.

The text in bold are names of the volume on that layer. In this case, **9712:ANGIO...1-1label** refers to the label map. **9712:ANGIO...e-scale_1** would be the DICOM dataset.

4- Co-ordinates in the bracket reflect the position of the pointer on the slice. Each slice in each orientation has its own set of co-ordinates, with origins starting from top left corner of the slice.

5- The last digits in bold refers to the value of the exact pixel the mouse pointer is on. The value can range from **-1000** (black) to over **3000** (almost white). We can then choose a suitable threshold range when we are fine-tuning the label map.

For label maps, the values are either **0 (0)** or **1 (1)**. These are the only values Model Maker recognizes.

3.8 Patching the label map (Wand Effect)

The **Wand Effect** is very effective as it works through multiple slices in a relatively short time. Adding Threshold range increases its precision

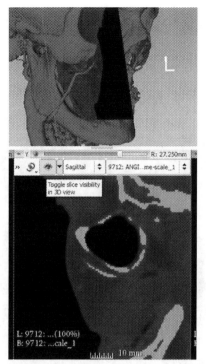

Mouse over the pin icon on the top left corner in slice view. A bar drops down, giving you extra options and information.

Hitting the eye icon toggles visibility of the slice in the 3D viewport above.

This ensures that you know the exact region you are working on when patching the label map within the slice viewer.

Figure 40 Displaying the slice in 3D space

As you move through the slices, the position of the slice updates in 3D view live.

You can have all 3 orientations visible in the 3D viewport at the same time

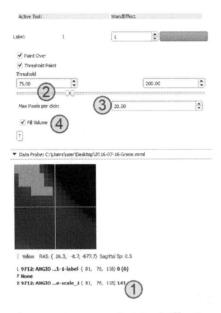

Figure 41 Setting up the **Wand Effect**

1- Choose a median spot on the slice viewer and get its value. (**141** in this case)

2- Set the threshold range to base on the value you got below, giving a buffer on both ends.

3- Set the **Max Pixels per click** to suit the situation. 20 is low in this case because the area is relatively small.

4- Turn on the **Fill Volume** option so we can work with multiple slices at once

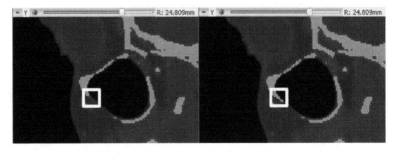

Figure 42 First pass of **Wand Effect**

On the right, all the pixels within our defined threshold range, that are connected, are selected. (In the white box) This effect permeates through the slices. Click a few times on the same spot until the area stops growing.

Use the same threshold setting and go through the other regions and layers to add as much areas within the range as possible.

Adjust the threshold range accordingly, to fill all the other areas. It will be extremely useful to have a good image reference by your side if you are not familiar with the anatomy of the region.

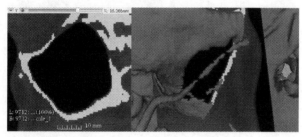

In a few minutes of work with the **Wand Effect** tool, we have roughly filled the gap in the maxilla bone.

Figure 43 Patched up hole

The label map on the 3d viewport updates live, making it easier to visualize your progress.

3.9 Patching the label map (Manual painting)

To polish up the edges, you may use the **Paint Effect**, **Draw Effect** and **Erase Label** tools.

Take note that it might be easier to turn off **Threshold Paint** on the **Paint Effect**. You are now manually painting the label map. Having a threshold applied over your paint strokes might yield undesirable results.

Use 'z' or 'y' key to **Undo** and **Redo** previous steps respectively. If you are using a stylus pen to paint the label map, you can move between slices with the arrow keys. Otherwise, the mouse roller works the same.

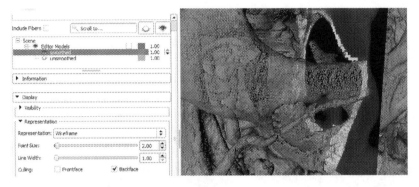

Figure 44 Achieving a see-through effect

While working on the outer surface of the model is intuitive, the interior organic forms on the skull can be difficult to visualize. We can exploit the display properties under the **Models** module to achieve an 'X-ray' view of the model.

Under the **Representation** sub-tab, change the representation type to **Wireframe**. As shown in *Figure 44*, this allows you to see through the exterior surface, while maintaining the distinction between the exterior surfaces and the interior.

Changing the color of the model to contrast against the color of your label map also helps you visualize your progress better.

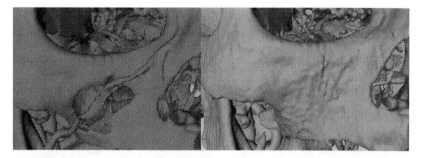

Figure 45 Comparing the result of the patch

It is advisable that you do a render with **Make Model** to check your progress once in a while to see how your patch looks like.

In *Figure 45*, we can see that the hole is patched up, but the surface is not as smooth. This is typical of a manual patch work, but is not a big issue. We can smooth it out later when preparing it for printing.

3.10 Saving and loading your progress

While it is easy to manage the 3D models from the **Models** module, saving and loading your label map is not as direct as it may seem.

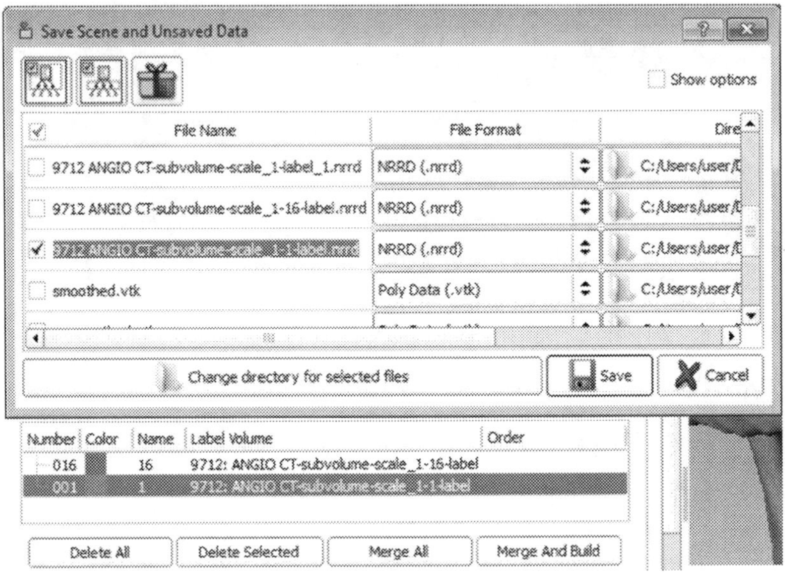

Figure 46 Identifying the Label Map to save

Click on the Save Data button to bring up the **Save Scene and Unsaved Data** window. Look for the .nrrd file that corresponds to the name of your label map.

Make sure you have saved your scene before this, and that you set the directory to a folder that is easy to locate.

Do not rename the .nrrd file. This will save only the label map of interest.

Next, we will learn how to set up an incremental save system within the work folder. This will be useful in case you make mistakes when patching your label map, and run out of **Undo** instances.

Please follow the steps closely as there is a potential risk of losing all your progress.

1- Save your entire scene in a work folder. I name mine **'Segmentation'**.

2- Create **'Incremental Saves'** and **'Back Ups'** folder in the main folder.

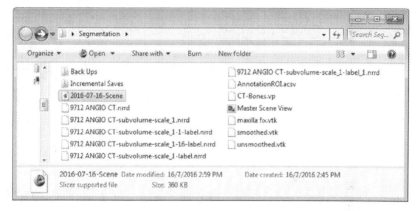

Figure 47 Creating **'Back Ups'** and **'Incremental Saves'** folders

3- To make an incremental save, click on the **Save Data** button, select only the label map of interest. Change its directory to the **'Incremental Saves'** folder. You may rename this file for easy recognition later.

Once you chose the directory, hit **Save**. **'incremental save 1.nrrd'** will be saved into **'Incremental Saves'** folder.

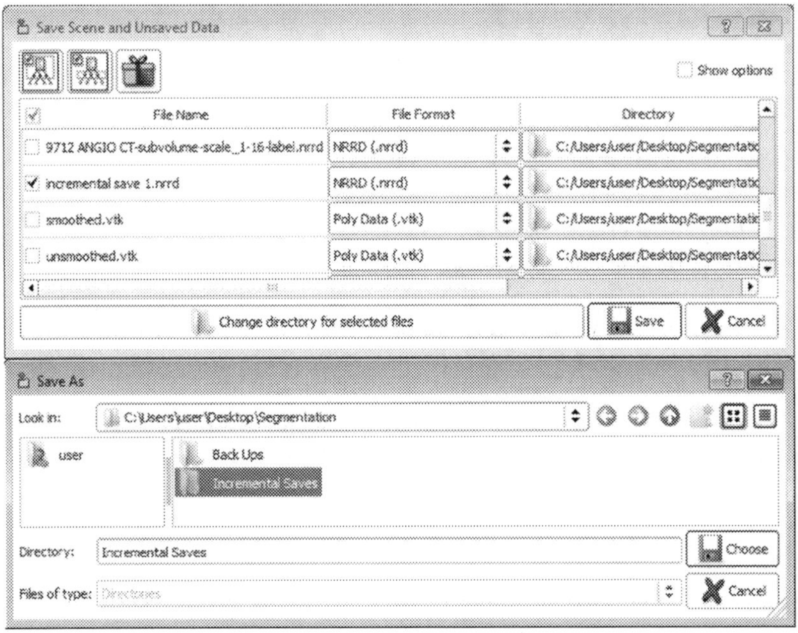

Figure 48 Saving the **Label Map** in 'Incremental Saves' folder

Note: *Make you change the directory back to the main work folder the next time you save your scene.*

It is recommended that you make an incremental save before exploring a new area of area of interest. Saving your data is encouraged in different stages of patching.

4- If there you have made mistakes in patching and run out of **Undo** options, you can always return to your last incremental save.

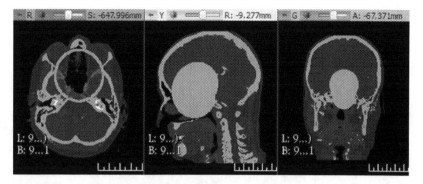

Figure 49 Running out of undo options after making a mistake

5- Save your scene and close it.

6- Go to your working folder and locate the label map file. In this case, '**9712 ANGIO CT-subvolume-scale_1-1-label**'.

7- Move the file into the '**Back Ups**' folder.

8- Locate the instance that you wish to roll back to from the incremental saves. (Refer to the time stamp on the file.)

9- Copy that file into '**Segmentation**' folder.

10- Rename it exactly like the original label map file.

The idea is to replace the label map file with older versions of itself. When you reopen the scene, 3D slicer loads the older label map, restoring your progress.

This is unconventional, but it will save you a lot of grief when you mess up the label map; especially when working on a particularly tedious segmentation.

3.11 Exporting the model

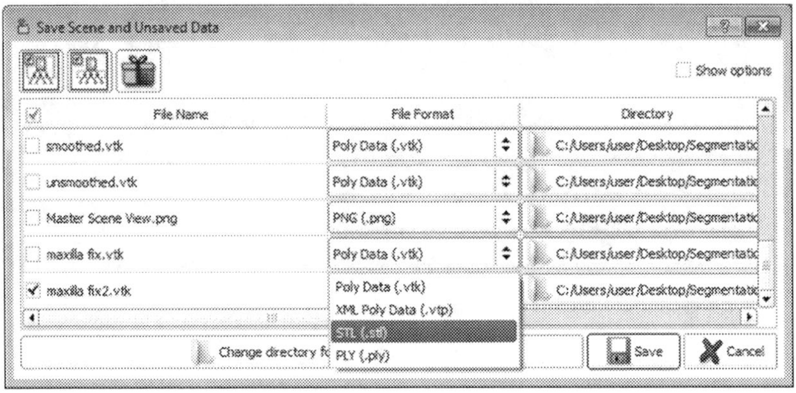

Figure 50 Saving the model as .stl

After patching up all the possible areas, we are ready to export the model. Do not worry if certain areas seem impossible to patch within 3D slicer. We will discuss solutions in chapter 4.Click **Save Data**. In the **Save Scene and Unsaved Data** window, look for the model you want to export, check on that item. Change its file format to **STL (.stl)**, and **Save**.

The save directory and file name will be on default, you may change them as you like.

This saves the model as an .stl (STereoLithography) file. This file format is supported by many other 3D software packages and is widely used for rapid prototyping and 3D printing.

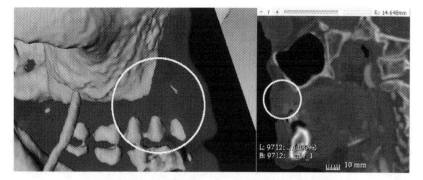

Figure 51 An area that is difficult to patch due to unclear dataset

Conclusion

Depending on the quality of your dataset, certain areas can be very difficult to segment due to the limitations on the imaging device. In *Figure 51*, the alveolar processes are largely nonexistent. From analyzing the dataset, we see that the bone masses did not show up like the other regions and therefore impossible for 3D Slicer's algorithms to pick up.

It is almost impossible, labor-intensive and inaccurate to segment it manually in 3D slicer.

The model generated can only be as good as the dataset. Every medical imaging system has its own limitations. Different regions of the body require different imaging techniques. Consequently, other regions might turn up fuzzy in the dataset.

There is no one universal algorithm that will work on all medical images, often, not even between different regions of the same dataset. Each dataset will come with its own set of limitations and flaws, and thus, each segmentation should be approached differently.

While there might be many extensions in the Module list (even more you can download under Extension Manager (**Ctrl + 4**)) to solve some common problems; the goal of this tutorial is to help you understand the fundamental relationship between the label map, and the 3D model.

Finally, please kindly note that the segmentation method discussed thus far is for research and educational purposes only. The application of this workflow is **NOT** recommended for clinical usage or for the design of medical devices.

CHAPTER 4

Other Tools

Exploring other tools

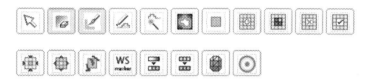

Figure 52 A look at other tools

In the previous chapter, we discussed some basic tools commonly used, and how your label map is translated to the 3D model; we now look at some other tools that can speed up the segmentation process.

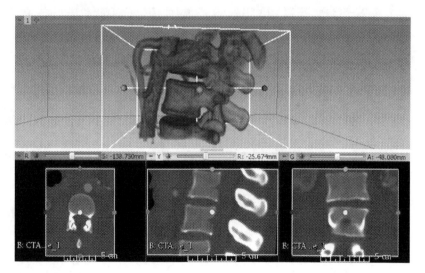

Figure 53 Isolating the vertebral columns

Let us pick up from where we left off. I will explain the functions of the remaining tools through another example.

For this tutorial, I will attempt to segment the two vertebral columns with the help of the remaining tools. This dataset (**CTA cardio**) can be downloaded under the **Sample Data** module.

4.1 Identify Island Effect:

The algorithm identifies islands of connected regions on your label map and gives it unique label. Connected regions are groups of voxels that are in contact with each other at a point, edge or face. Groups of voxels that only share faces are considered **Fully Connected**.

Voxels are what the mesh of the model is built upon. Think 3D pixels.

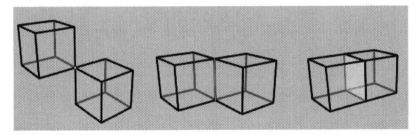

Figure 54 From left: Voxels connected at a Point, Edge and Face

We begin by applying a **Threshold Effect** over the dataset. Adjust the threshold setting to find the sweet spot, and Apply.

Active Tool: IdentifyIslandsEffect

Label: 1 | 1   ⏷ | ▓▓▓▓▓▓▓

☑ Fully Connected
Minimum Size
| 0   ⏷ |
| Apply |

Figure 55 Identify Island Effect properties

The settings are simple. Label defines which color you want the algorithm to analyze. Checking **Fully Connected** tell the function to only consider fully connected voxels.

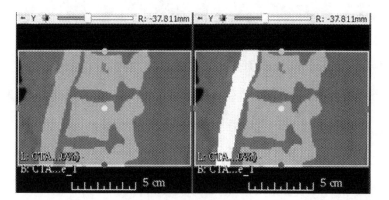

Figure 56 After applying **Identify Island Effect**

After applying **Identify Island Effect**, we see that the region that defines the aorta artery is highlighted with a different color, while the rest remains the same. The operation assigns labels from the list on the color table that you picked from the start. Starting from the largest volume.

Note: *If your segmentation is not clean (with a lot of floating islands), using this tool will generate too many structures, and slow down the processor.*

The top vertebrae and the bottom vertebrae are assigned the same label. If you scroll down the slices, you will find that they are still connected at certain areas.

This tool works best on areas with well-defined edges.

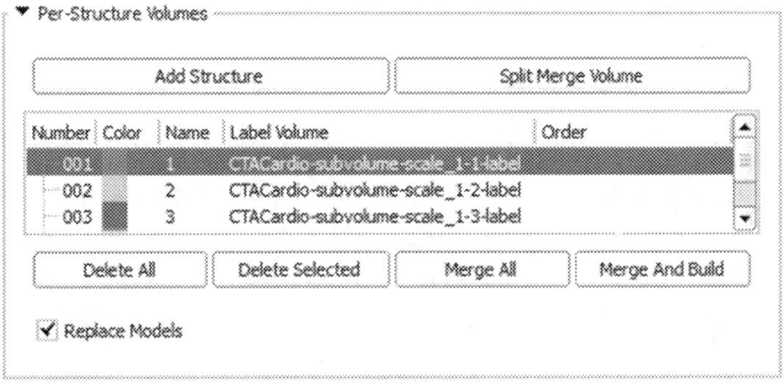

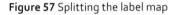

Figure 57 Splitting the label map

Under the Per-Structure Volumes sub-tab, click on the Split Merge Volume to split it into individual labels. We can now use the label map that contains the vertebrae bones to create our model.

4.2 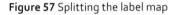 Change Island Effect:

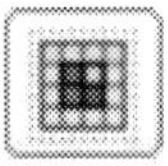

The Change Island Effect tool work very much like the Identify Island Effect. In this, you manually select the group of voxels that you want to re-label. The advantage of this is that, unlike its automated counterpart, you can be specific about the island you want to re-label. In the example from *Figure 57*, I ended up with over 200 different structures when I split the merge volume.

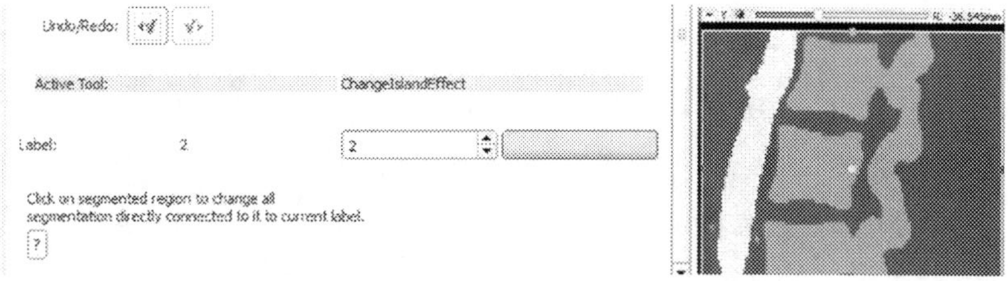

Figure 58 Assigning label '**2**' to the aorta artery

1- Set the new label that you want assign.

2- Click on the region on the Slice Viewer to Change its label.

Similarly, we can split the merge volume into individual structure.

This tool is useful when you need to isolate individual islands, while keeping the others intact.

4.3 **Remove Islands Effect:**

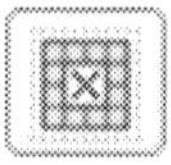

This tool identifies the largest group of voxels as the main region and removes other smaller regions that are not connected or loosely connected to it.

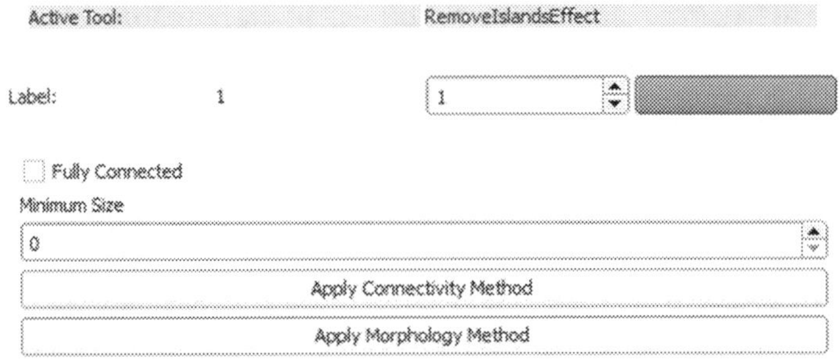

Active Tool: RemoveIslandsEffect

Label: 1   1

☐ Fully Connected
Minimum Size
0

Apply Connectivity Method

Apply Morphology Method

Figure 59 Remove Island Effect properties

Label defines the label map of interest. The Fully Connected option works exactly as mentioned above. Below are two way to remove islands in different circumstances.

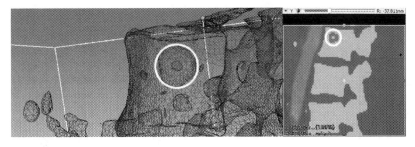

Figure 60 Apply Connectivity Method removes holes within segmented areas (Circled in white)

Apply Connectivity Method: This method removes empty areas that are enclosed within segmented areas. Using this mode, we can quickly remove holes created within a model due to the difference in density from the dataset.

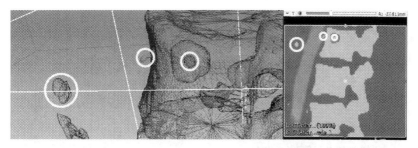

Figure 61 Apply morphology Method removes noise segments (Circled in white)

Apply Morphology method: This method removes small islands that are not part of, or loosely connected to the segmentation, even if they are inside the empty pockets within it. This tool allows you to quickly remove noise from your segmentation. Very helpful when cleaning up a particularly fuzzy dataset.

4.4 Save Island Effect:

Save Island retains the region that you select, and removes all other unconnected islands. Another quick and easy method to clean up your segmentation.

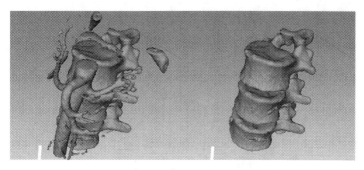

Figure 62 Before and after applying Save Island Effect

4.5 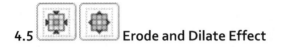 Erode and Dilate Effect

These two effects are the exact opposite of each other. Erode removes a layer of pixels on the selected label while Dilate adds. These can be quite useful for clean up when applied correctly with **Remove Islands Effect.**

There are two options for this operation, **Eight Neighbors** and **Four Neighbors**. They simply mean how much to add or remove.

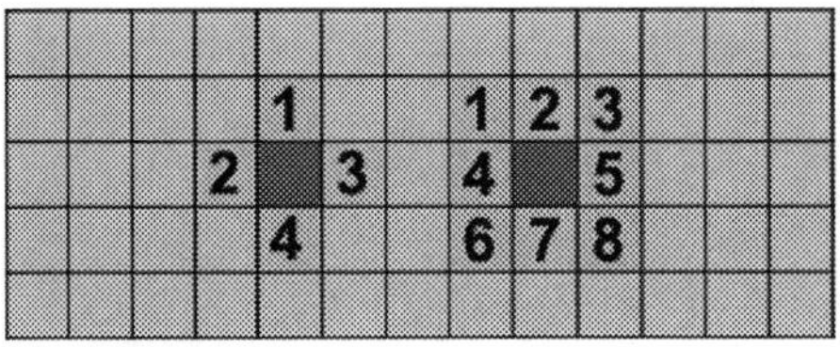

Figure 63 Pixel connectivity

I will not go into details about pixel neighborhood. *Figure 63* illustrates the difference between four and eight neighbors.

4.6 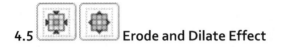 Grow Cut and Watershed from Markers Effect

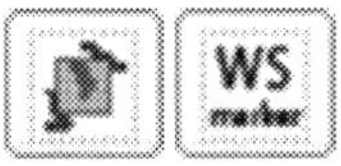

These two are very powerful tools and yields similar results. First you draw markings on the region that you want to extract. Then, with another color, draw on the outside of the region of interest.

The algorithms samples whatever you have marked and identifies the edge of the segmentation. The more information you provide it to work with, the better the result will be, so try to put your markings on multiple slices and through multiple layers. Also, try to include the range of values within the segmentation with your markings.

Note: *The process can take some time to complete, have some patience, and save your progress before you hit **Apply**.*

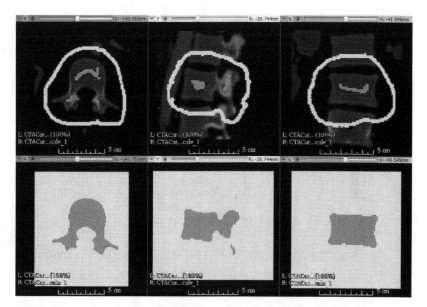

Figure 64 Using **Grow Cut/ Watershed from Markers Effect**

These tools give a clean segmentation in a very short amount of time, with minimal effort; provided, the dataset itself is of good quality.

4.7 Change Label Effect

Changes all the voxels within a label that corresponds to the input level into the output level.

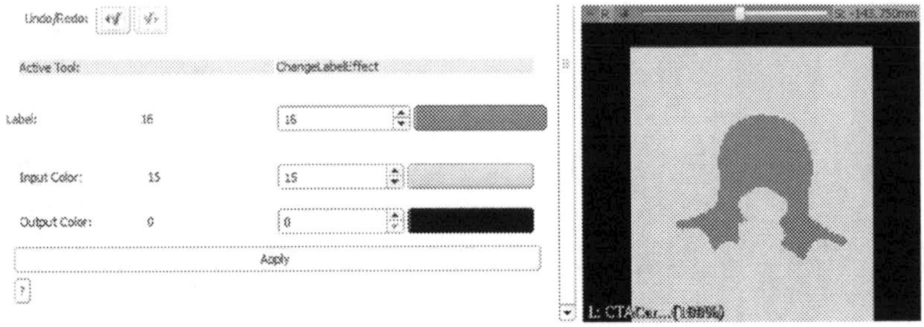

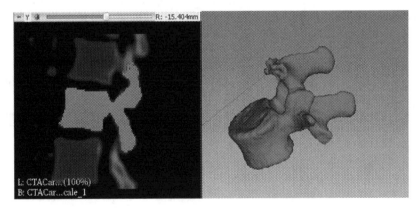

Figure 65 Changing color '**15**' to '**0**'

Choose the color that you want to change from **Input Color**. You can get the number of the color from the **Data Probe** tab if you are unsure.

The **Output Color** option defines the color that you want to change it into. '0' removes the selection. Which in this case is exactly our intention.

Figure 66 Achieving very fast results with **Grow Cut/ Watershed from Markers**, plus **Change Label** tools

A look at what we can do with the more advanced tools in under five minutes. We have illuminated all the noise, and achieved a relatively good segmentation. Of course this is not perfect. To remove the spinous process of the vertebrae above, we can either go in with **Erase Effect** to clean up, or go back and place more markers in the problem region to generate the better result. Either way, it will not take much effort.

4.8 ◉ Fast Marching Effect

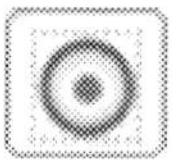

Fast marching works similar to **Grow Cut** and **Watershed from Markers** effects, but only uses one color. You paint in the area of interest to define sample voxels. The algorithm grows the label with the sample data.

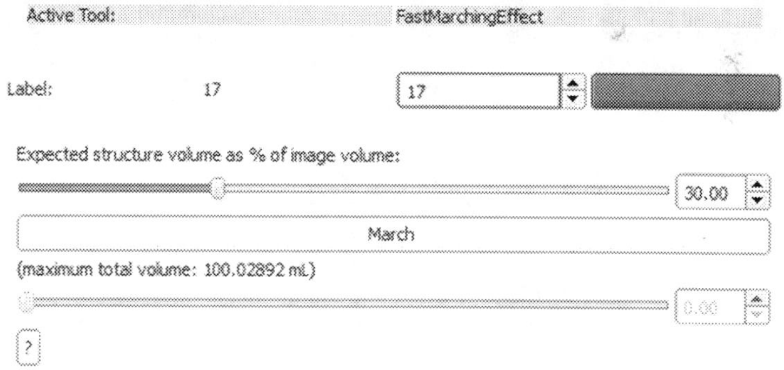

Active Tool:		FastMarchingEffect	
Label:	17	17	

Expected structure volume as % of image volume:

30.00

March

(maximum total volume: 100.02892 mL)

0.00

Figure 67 Fast Marching Effect properties

Expected structure volume as % of image volume: slider assigns the amount of growth before you run the algorithm.

(Maximum total volume :) slider controls the amount of growth after you have run the algorithm.

You may run as many marches as you like to get your results. In between marches, you can go in and edit out the areas that strayed out of boundaries.

Note: *This tool works well on regions with consistent density and clear boundary.*

The aorta artery seems like a good region to use this tool on first look, due to its consistency reflected on the dataset.

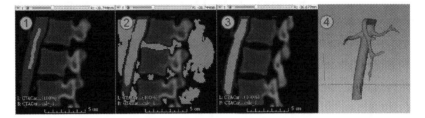

Figure 68 Segmenting the aorta artery with **Fast Marching**

1- Drawing on the region to mark out samples.

2- Applying the **Fast March**.

3- Toning it down with **Maximum Total Volume** control and manually editing out small stray regions.

4- After repeating steps 2 and 3 a few times, we can see that the result is a clean segmentation.

As with **Grow Cut** and **Watershed from Markers**, providing it with more sample data to work with yields better results. By spending a little more time to mark out small areas that the algorithm might have trouble reaching, we can achieve quite an accurate segmentation.

Moving on...

With all the above tools, we should be able to achieve a decent segmentation. Now we are finally ready to move on and prepare it for 3D printing.

CHAPTER 5

Preparing for printing

5.1 Introduction to Autodesk Meshmixer

Meshmixer is a free software by Autodesk, and is widely used for 3D printing. We could use any 3D platforms available out there to edit our segmentation, but we find Meshmixer to be quick and easy to use as while it is built to facilitate 3D printing. The software also includes many tools and function to help us edit and prepare our segmentation for printing.

Previously we encountered many issues when segmenting the skull. Now let us take a look at how Meshmixer can help resolve some of the problems we faced.

Some problems are easier solved in 3D slicer, while others in Meshmixer. It all depends on the situation. With experience, you will be able to access the situation and plan your work flow from analyzing the DICOM dataset with **Volume Render.**

5.2 User interface

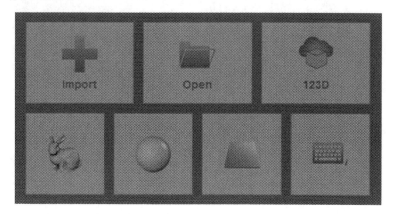

Figure 69 Prompt window on startup

On startup, you will be prompted with the above icons. Choose Import, and locate the .stl file of the skull that we exported from 3D slicer.

For this tutorial we will only go through some of it many tools and functions that we need. A full documentation of the software is available on its official website.

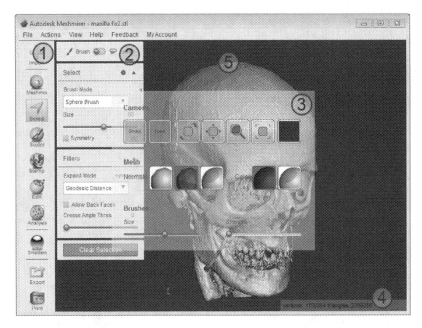

Figure 70 Meshmixer standard UI

1- **Toolbar:** A list of common tools. (Sculpt, Stamp, Edit, etc.)

2- **Tool property**: Opens up when you select a tool. Displays tool properties and sub-tools.

3- **Hotbox**: Hold **Spacebar** to display **Camera**, **Mesh** and **Brush** option.

4- Displays statistics of the selected model.

5- Navigating the **work space**.

- ('**Alt**' + **Left mouse button** + drag)/ (**Right mouse button** + drag)/ ('**Shift**' + **Middle mouse button** + drag): Rotate view

- **Middle mouse button**: Move camera

- **Middle mouse roller**: Zoom in/out

- '**c**': Centers the camera to mouse pointer

- '(**'**/ ')': Redo/ Undo camera movement

- '**w**': Toggle display wireframe

- '**Shift**' + '**v**': Toggle visibility of selected object

- '**Ctrl**' + '**Shift**' + '**v**': Show all objects

- '**Ctrl**' + '**Shift**' + '**v**': Toggle object window

5.3 Reducing the triangle count

Models generated by Make Model Effect usually have a very high triangle count. We will start by reducing it so that the scene runs more smoothly.

1- Activate the Select tool (press '**s**'), dial the brush size down to a single digit.

2- Double click on the model to select the entire island. Double click on other regions to add selections.

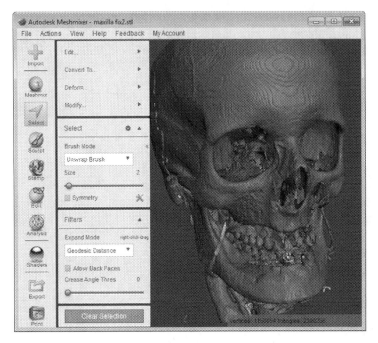

Figure 71 Skull selected appears in a different color

3- Press 'i' to invert selection.

4- Press 'x' to delete.

This gets rid of the noise in the scene. Before you delete unwanted volumes, do check thoroughly that you do not delete any regions that you need.

Press 'w' to display the wireframe. Right now, the wireframe is very dense, and the scene might be sluggish due to the heavy model.

While using the **Edit> Remesh** function can reduce the triangle count automatically, it is not effective at this point.

'**Remesh**' is unpredictable and takes too long to process. Most importantly, it applies the same level to mesh reduction across the entire model, potentially eliminating some details in the process.

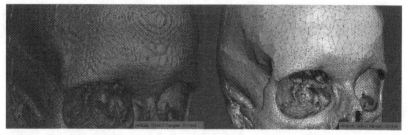

Figure 72 Reducing the triangle count manually

It is more advisable manually reduce the triangle at this point.

1- Go to **Sculpt> Brushes> RobustSmooth**

2- Under **Properties** tab, set **Strength** to **0**, **Size** to **50**

3- Under **Refine** tab, check **Enable Refine**. Set **Reduce** to whatever value best suits the level of details you need (Figure72, Reduce= 40 for cranium, Reduce= 20 for orbital bones) and all others to **0**.

4- Paint over the surface of the model to reduce the triangles. In the example, we managed to reduce the triangle count by 90%, which still maintaining the important details.

With a lower triangle count, the scene is easier to work with.

5.4 Plane cut

In this segmentation, our region of interest is the cross section of the skull. So we have to cut it in half.

We prefer to do the cut in **Meshmixer**, over just doing a cross section segmentation of the skull from the get go. While is it fine to do the cut in 3d Slicer, the problem with **Make Model** is that it will smooth out even the sliced edge, leaving a fuzzy edge. This is undesirable, especially when you want both sides to be able to fit together after you print it out.

Furthermore, doing the cut prior to triangle reduction will cause further deterioration of the edge. Cutting of the model should be done once you have reduced the triangle sufficiently throughout the model.

Plane cut allows you to define a plane to cut the model at. It leaves the clean, sharp edge, with the option to close up the holes left from the cut.

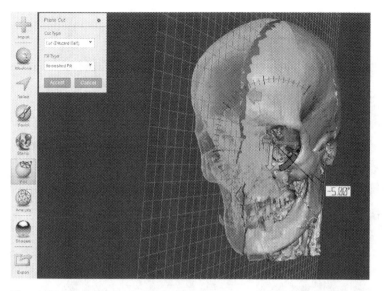

Figure 73 Adjusting the cutting angle. Translucent half will be deleted (**Cut (Discard Half)**).

1- Go to **Edit> Plane Cut**.

2- A plane appears, with colored handles in the middle. Click and drag the arrows to transform in the respective directions. Drag the triangle to free transform, and the curve to rotate. While in rotate mode, move your cursor over the circular angle snap to exact angles.

3- In the **Plane Cut** properties tab, define the type of cut and fill.

Once you have to cut the model, if you choose **Slice (Keep Both)**, it will still be taken as a single entity. Double click to select one half. Go to **Edit> Edit> Separate** or hit the '**y**' key to split it into two objects.

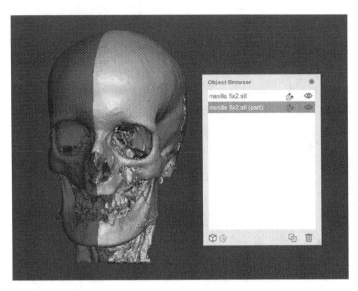

Figure 74 Splitting the cut model pieces into 2 separate objects

5.5 Further cleaning

Besides isolated islands, there are also unwanted mesh that are stuck to the main model. Follow these steps to quickly get rid of them.

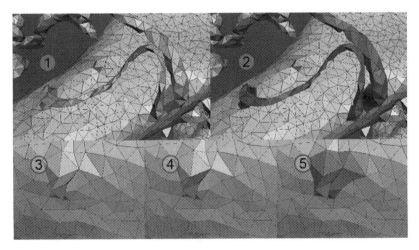

Figure 75 Cleaning islands that are joined to the main body

1- Select the ring of triangles around the base where the noise is joined to the main model. Press '**x**' to delete those faces.

2- Now that the noise is separated from the model, we can select the entire mass and delete them.

3- For minor bumps and dimples on the surface. Select the triangle in the middle.

4- Press '**<**' or '**>**' to expand or reduce one layer of selection. This works like **Erode** and **Dilate** in 3D slicer.

5- Grow the selection towards the boundaries and delete the faces.

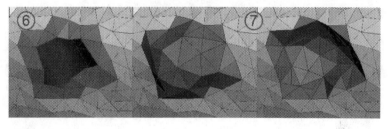

Figure 76 Fill hole

6- Double click on any triangle that has an edge in the boundary of the hole to select the entire ring.

7- Use the **Scale** and **Bulge** to control the surface of the fill.

The **Refine** slider determines the mesh density of the area being filled.

5.6 Fixing flaws from the segmentation

We have previously discussed how to fix the hole in the maxilla bone in 3D slicer. There are tools in Meshmixer that can do similar job. The advantage of Meshmixer lies in the interactive aspect. You are able to control the amount of details you give to the fix and see the effect of your patch live.

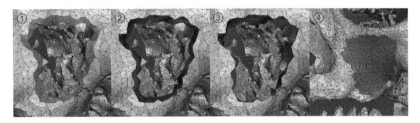

Figure 77 Fixing the flaw in the segmentation

1- Paint a selection of ring around the hole. Make sure all the triangles are connected in at least one edge.

2- Delete the ring.

3- Double click to select the interior ring, use '>' to expand the selection if needed. Delete the ring to get rid of the triangles that makes up the thickness of the hole.

4- Fill the hole and set the bulge/dent to fit the curvature of the surface. Do the same for the whole created at the back.

To get a more accurate fix, it is better to use an anatomical reference. Fixing the model this way is only for meant aesthetic purposes, we do not recommend using the result for any medical applications.

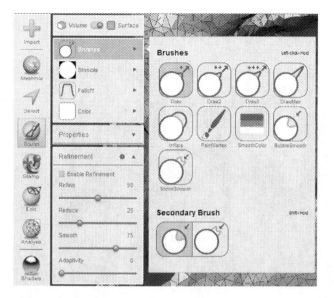

Figure 78 Seleceting sculpting brushes

After filling in the holes, we can use the **Sculpt** too to add in anatomical details.

1- Change brush setting to **Surface**.

2- Go to **Sculpt> Brushes**, choose the **Draw** brush, and **BubbleSmooth** as secondary brush.

3- Set the **Strength** and **Size** to suit your need.

4- Uncheck the **Enable Refinement**.

5- Paint on the surface to add volume, hold `Ctrl` to apply reduce.

Use `[` or `]` to change the size of your brush.

Although you may use the Refine tool to add mesh to your area of interest if needed.

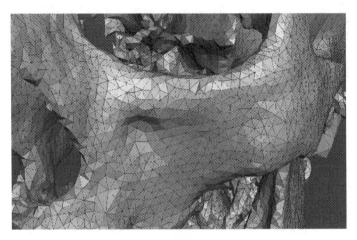

Figure 79 Adding anatomical details with Sculpt

5.7 Bridging gaps

When two islands are not physically joined, we can use the Bridge tool to join it back.

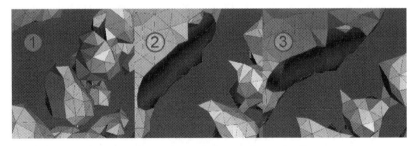

Figure 80 Opening up holes on islands to bridge them with the main volume

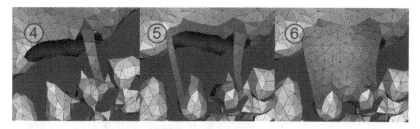

Figure 81 Bridging the island, and filling the hole

1- As per previously mentioned, select areas of the mesh that you need to cut open.

2- Delete triangles to create an opening to **bridge**.

3- On both sides of the islands, select triangles to merge.

4- Press '**Ctrl**' + '**b**' to bridge. You may choose more than one triangle on each side to bridge.

5- On another end of the gap, perform another bridge to create an enclosed area.

6- Fill the hole, and use the **Refine** slider to increase the density as needed.

Go on and bridge all other areas, including the back of the teeth.

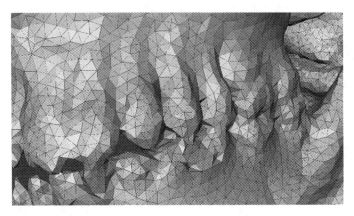

Figure 82 Merging the teeth back with the main volume

With a bit more time, we can add in the missing details.

4.8 Preparing for print

With the model cleaned up and flaws fixed, we are ready to perform our last preparations for printing.

We will create a base for the model, align and scale it.

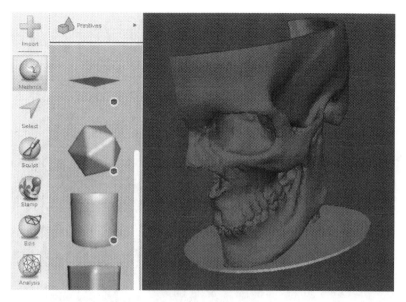

Figure 83 Using a default basic shape for the base

To create a base for the model, go to **Meshmix**.

Under **Primitives** tab, click and drag the cylinder into the 3D scene.

Using the handles, scale and move it under the model. Make sure the models slightly intersect.

To combine them into a single entity, select both together under the **Object Browser** window.

Under **Edit**, select **Boolean Union**.

Make sure there are no whole on the surface of the union. If Boolean Union causes deformation on either object, we can use the **remesh** method to add density to the contact surfaces. **Boolean Union** works better on surfaces with similar mesh density.

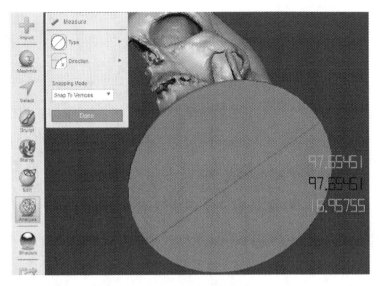

Figure 84 Measuring the diameter of the base

Under the **Analysis> Measure** tool, use the measuring tools to measure the scale of your model.

Use the transform option to rescale your model. You can manually enter a scale value to get an exact measurement.

Toggle the visibility of the Printer Bed under the **View** tab.

Use the **Align** and **Transform** function under the **Edit** tool to align the model to the printer bed.

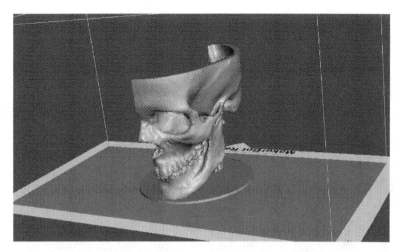

Figure 85 Aligning the model to the base of the print bed

Before we can print, we should do a last check for any errors. Use the Inspector tool under the Analysis tab to diagnose the model for any errors. Then use the Auto Repair function to troubleshoot.

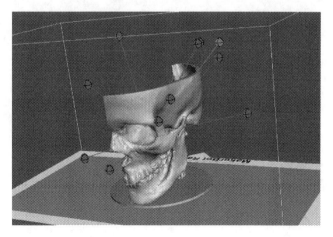

Figure 86 Inspector detects errors on the model

The last step is to export the model. Select the final model, and export it as .stl to be print-ready.

CHAPTER 6

Conclusion

We hope you now have a basic understanding of the process of segmentation, and how it translates to a 3D model.

There are myriad methods and programs out there that can produce the same results. However, the workflow process that we have introduced is simple, straight forward and available free. It is suitable for beginners to kick start their journey into 3D printing.

For the beginners, the 3D slicer may appear overwhelming initially due to the numerous modules, controls and range sliders. However, it is essential that you spend some time to get comfortable with the program. Practice makes perfect. Having a good grasp on the workings of 3D slicer enables you to make a smooth transition to other commercial programs. Most other segmentation programs are built on the same concept.

As for cleaning up with Meshmixer, we find that the software hits the sweet spot for our needs. While virtually any 3D software can perform the same job, most are not built for this purpose. Furthermore, any new user will be overwhelmed since these other programs are more complicated and sophisticated to handle than the 3D slicer and Meshmixer put together.

Now that you have the foundation, we hope you will continue to explore the wonders of 3D printing of medical models

Yihua Li, Eric Luis

6.1 Acknowledgements

3D slicer is a free open source software distributed under a BSD style license. All use and mention of the software within this publication falls within fair use.

The DICOM dataset '**MANIX**' belongs to Pixmeo (A swiss company specialized in medical imaging software development and PACS installation support). The owners of Pixmeo has kindly granted us permission to use their dataset in this publication.

Meshmixer is the 'Swiss Army Knife' for 3D meshes. All use and mention of the software within this publication complies with their software license agreements.